VITAMIN E—A PROTECTIVE FORCE

For decades accepted as merely an antioxidant, vitamin E's capacities have been increasingly recognized until it is now firmly established as a protective force in natural therapy. It is used by surgeons before and after operations to ensure against thrombosis and increase immunity to infection, by pediatricians to prevent blindness in premature babies and by other specialists to increase high density lipoproteins. It decreases elevated hormone levels and prevents and treats anemias and cystic breast disease. Vitamin E has just begun to act. This Guide brings you up to date on one of the most vital nutrients of them all.

ABOUT THE AUTHOR AND EDITORS

Len Mervyn, Ph.D., is a chartered chemist and fellow of the Royal Institute of Chemistry in England. He taught at Ewell College of Advanced Technology in Surrey and now works for Booker Health Foods Ltd. as technical director. Dr. Mervyn's work with vitamin B12 earned him awards from the New York Academy of Sciences and from the University of Pavia in Italy. He has written many books on biochemistry and nutrition including *Minerals and Your Health* and *Chelated Mineral Nutrition in Plants, Animals and Man*.

Richard A. Passwater, Ph.D., is one of the most called-upon authorities for information relating to preventive health care. A noted biochemist, he is credited with popularizing the term "supernutrition" largely as a result of having written two bestsellers on the subject—*Supernutrition: Megavitamin Revolution* and *Supernutrition for Healthy Hearts*. His other books include *Easy No-Flab Diet*, *Cancer and Its Nutritional Therapies* and *Selenium as Food & Medicine*. He has just completed a new book, *Trace Elements, Hair Analysis and Nutrition* with Elmer M. Cranton, M.D.

Earl Mindell, R.Ph., Ph.D., combines the expertise and working experience of a pharmacist with extensive knowledge in most of the nutrition areas. His book *Earl Mindell's Vitamin Bible* is now a million-copy bestseller; and his more recent *Vitamin Bible for Your Kids* may very well duplicate his first *Bible's* publishing history. Dr. Mindell's popular *Quick & Easy Guide to Better Health* was published by Keats Publishing.

VITAMIN E UPDATED
NEW ROLES FOR THE VITAMIN THAT PRESERVES THE HEALTH AND INTEGRITY OF BODY CELLS

by Len Mervyn, Ph.D.

Keats Publishing, Inc.　　New Canaan, Connecticut

Vitamin E Updated is not intended as medical advice. Its intention is solely informational and educational. Please consult a medical or health professional should the need for one be warranted.

VITAMIN E UPDATED

Copyright © 1983 by Keats Publishing, Inc.

All Rights Reserved

No part of this book may be copied or reproduced in any form without the written consent of the publisher.

ISBN: 0-87983-274-6

Printed in the United States of America

Good Health Guides are published by Keats Publishing, Inc.
27 Pine Street (Box 876)
New Canaan, CT 06840

Contents

	Page
Introduction	1
How Vitamin E Functions	2
Vitamin E as a Protective Force	5

    The Prevention of Thrombosis
    Atherosclerosis
    Thrombophlebitis

Vitamin E as a Therapeutic Agent	15

    Anemia
    The Prevention of Blindness in Babies
    Cystic Breast Disease
    Resistance to Disease

New Insight into Vitamin E Potency	22
References	25

INTRODUCTION

It is now some sixty years since vitamin E was discovered and characterized, yet its functions, and even more its therapeutic uses, are still controversial in the scientific and medical fraternities. There are only three special situations where it is generally accepted that supplementary vitamin E has proved to be beneficial.

The first is in treating hemolytic anemia in newborn infants. Vitamin E is not actively transported from the maternal to the fetal circulation and it is poorly absorbed by those infants whose gestational age is less than thirty-six weeks. A deficiency of tocopherol (vitamin E) causes hemolytic anemia and widespread edema, two conditions that are reversed by vitamin E treatment.

The second is in treating deficiencies caused by the malabsorption of fats and oils since vitamin E is an oil.

Cystic fibrosis is invariably associated with vitamin E deficiency. Di Sant'Agnese's group at Bethesda (1977) has shown that most nonsupplemented patients suffering from cystic fibrosis are so deficient in vitamin E that their red blood cells are inadequately protected against oxidative stresses. Other conditions giving rise to malabsorption of fats and oils with subsequent vitamin E deficiency include liver cirrhosis, obstructive jaundice, pancreatic insufficiency and sprue. H. J. Binder and H. M. Shapiro (1967) studied patients with malabsorption problems and vitamin E deficiency and were able to relate this deficiency to the patients' long-term inability to absorb fats.

A study of any modern medical textbook will indicate that the only accepted therapy with vitamin E for a condition unrelated to fat absorption is for the treatment of intermittent claudication. This represents the third situation. Intermittent claudication is the term for calf pains when walking. It is caused by a narrowing of the arteries supplying blood to the leg muscles. The restricted blood supply gives rise to pain as the muscles become starved of oxygen. There are many publications in the world's medical press confirming the excellent response of this condition to vitamin E. Typical is that of K. Haeger (1974) who performed a double-blind study to show the benefits of vitamin E in this condition. The treatment requires 400 mg or more of vitamin E daily and therapy must continue for at least three months.

Over the last five or ten years we have become more aware of how vitamin E functions. This in turn has indicated how the vitamin might be used in treating certain clinical conditions whose etiology is related to abnormalities in those functions. The result is that it now looks likely that vitamin E may be beneficial in treating diseases in addition to those mentioned above. The evidence for such therapy will now be reviewed.

HOW VITAMIN E FUNCTIONS

In man, the only generally accepted role of vitamin E is a protective one, that of acting as an antioxidant in preserving the health and integrity of body cells and membranes. Biological membranes contain phospholipids and degradation of these by oxygen can cause loss of cell integrity. Phospholipids contain high quantities of polyunsaturated fatty acids (PUFA) and the double bonds of these acids are easily attacked by oxygen to produce the toxic fatty peroxides. The extent of formation of peroxides (i.e., peroxidation) increases with the number of double bonds in the fatty acids of the phospholipids, so membranes with a high PUFA content are especially likely to become oxidized. A common example of peroxidation is the rancidity of butter and vegetable oils. Vitamin E prevents this action of oxygen on the double bonds, possibly by inhibiting the enzyme catalyzing it, and so acts as a protective antioxidant.

Other agents produced both within and outside the body cells are the so-called free radicals. These substances are highly reactive because they are chemically incomplete and hence unstable, so they can latch onto other substances very readily. They are known also as superoxide radicals and they are produced within cells both by self-oxidation (as in peroxides) and by enzymative processes. Their high intrinsic reactivity and their ability to generate even more potent oxidizing agents when combined with peroxides constitute a constant threat to cellular integrity. Free radicals perform some useful functions, for example in the bactericidal action of white blood cells and in mediating the inflammatory response.

However, it is when they are produced in large quantity and their metabolic products allowed to go unchecked that they can seriously damage membranes and even denature DNA.

Since free radicals are continually being generated, the human body has developed a number of mechanisms to deal with their potentially damaging effects and those of their metabolites. The cellular defense mechanisms involve various enzymes such as superoxide dismutase, glutathione synthetase, glutathione peroxidase, glutathione reductase, glucose-6-phosphate, dehydrogenase and catalase. Plasma proteins with antioxidant potential include the copper-containing transferrin ceruloplasmin and the iron-containing transferrin. Food constituents that also contribute to protection include the sulphur-containing amino acids, the minerals selenium, zinc and copper and the vitamins riboflavin (vitamin B2) and tocopherol (vitamin E). The most widely studied protective agent in recent years, however, is vitamin E and it now looks as if this vitamin plays this key role, either directly or indirectly through the other agents. Ever since its discovery many clinical claims have been attributed to vitamin E. Now at last these empiric observations are finding a basis in sound biochemical functioning that places vitamin E firmly in an essential and established protective role.

The susceptibility of any tissue to an oxidative stress induced by free radicals or peroxide relates to the balance between the extent of that stress and the antioxidant ability of the protective agents. Where the tissue is genetically defective in its ability to provide protection, giving extra quantities of the protective agents can go part of the way in overcoming the defect. Hence, once we recognize the biological antioxidant property of vitamin E, it is possible to equate the conditions where it is beneficial to the doses required for efficacy.

First there are those conditions which relate to a simple deficiency state. These include the hemolytic anemia of low birth weight infants; the shortening of red blood cell life in those suffering from cystic fibrosis; the high tendency of blood platelets to aggregate in patients with biliary atresia; the lack of growth and brain dysfunctions that occur in a betalipoproteinemia where essential plasma lipoproteins are absent.

Second, there are those conditions where there is no evidence of deficiency of the vitamin but nevertheless large doses appear to prevent the effects of an oxidative assault. The prime example here is the success of vitamin E in preventing or reducing the severity of retrolental fibroplasia (producing blindness) in premature infants who have been exposed to high oxygen intake for the treatment of respiratory distress.

The third category includes conditions where frank pharmacological doses of the vitamin have been employed. There is no sign of a deficiency but there appears to be some preexisting defect in the body's defense mechanisms against free radicals. The diseases that respond are usually related to specific enzyme deficiencies and the common factor is a hemolytic anemia or sickle-cell anemia.

All the above categories relate to the action of vitamin E in protecting against excessive oxidation stress or free radical production. There are, however, also reports on how the vitamin has helped in overcoming blood vessel thromboses, blood platelet dysfunctions, atherosclerosis and breast tumors and cysts. It appears also to exert an influential effect upon the ability to resist infection (immune responses). Perhaps these benefits also relate to its antioxidant and protective role but the evidence is not clearcut. What we shall do now is to review critically the recent evidence that once more puts vitamin E into the forefront of natural therapy. At the same time our increasing knowledge of how vitamin E functions indicates why it may help in therapy and this too will be discussed.

VITAMIN E AS A PROTECTIVE FORCE

The prevention of thrombosis. Thrombosis is the formation of a thrombus, defined in medical dictionaries as a clot of blood formed within the heart or blood vessels, usually due to a slowing of the circulation or to alteration of the blood or vessel walls. The coronary arteries supply blood and hence oxygen to the heart muscle itself, allowing the organ to function effectively. There are two types of coronary heart disease: 1) that due to partial or total blockage of the artery by a blood clot (coronary thrombosis); and 2) that due to deposition of fats onto the artery wall (atherosclerosis), which also leads to constriction of the blood flow. Recent research indicates that vitamin E can help prevent and in some cases reverse these two conditions.

During the 1940s, the Shute brothers, in their practice in Canada, noted that vitamin E both dissolved fresh preformed blood clots and prevented their formation. They believed the vitamin exerted its action by inhibiting the protein thrombin which normally functions as a blood clot inducer. Normally this is a natural defense to prevent excessive bleeding when a blood vessel is damaged. However, sometimes the process gets out of hand and a thrombus forms for no apparent reason, with serious manifestations.

During the 1950s further studies were published in the *Journal of the American Medical Association* on the importance of vitamin E in dissolving and preventing blood clots. In 1964 Dr. Alton Ochsner and his group published confirmatory studies in the

New England Journal of Medicine and stated that "alpha tocopherol is a potent inhibitor of thrombin that does not produce excessive bleeding and is therefore a safe preventative agent against thrombosis."

Now studies reported in the late 1970s have given a clearer insight into how a thrombus is formed, how platelets, the tiny white blood cells, contribute to this, and how the whole process may be controlled. It now seems as if vitamin E plays a prominent part in preventing platelet aggregation.

The first thing that happens when a blood vessel wall is damaged is that the blood platelets collect around the affected area, change shape and form aggregates. Red blood cells become enmeshed in the platelet aggregate and thicken it. The cell aggregates in turn are held together by the precipitation from the blood plasma of the protein fibrin which forms a network. The final result is a large, stable thrombus which may eventually occlude the blood vessel.

What makes platelets aggregate is their stickiness and this in turn is controlled by certain hormones that are normally produced within the body. It is the production and balance of these hormones that determine the aggregation of platelets. They are known as prostaglandins and they in turn are influenced by vitamin E.

The material from which prostaglandins are made is an essential polyunsaturated fatty acid called arachidonic, itself manufactured from linoleic acid. This gives rise to an important hormone called prostacyclin, produced by the blood vessel walls. It is also released by the lungs and other tissues and acts in the blood, constantly preventing platelets from sticking to vessel walls. Prostacyclin is the most potent inhibitor of platelet aggregation known and it also acts as a vasodilator, i.e., keeps blood vessels open. However, from the same precursor, arachidonic acid, another hormone called thromboxane is produced. This is formed solely by the platelets and it has an action directly opposite that of prostacyclin. It causes platelets to aggregate and blood vessels to narrow; in other words it is a vasoconstrictor. Hence the stickiness of the platelets and the ability to form blood clots or thrombi depends on the balance between the opposite effects of prostacyclin and thromboxane. Both hormones are unstable, breaking down into inert compounds. Prostacyclin is the "good" hormone, thromboxane the "bad" one, and an imbalance in favor of thromboxane could well contribute to a heart attack or stroke.

We have seen that arachidonic acid is the precursor of both prostacyclin and thromboxane but at the same time there are alternative metabolic pathways for this highly unsaturated acid. It can be oxidized by an enzyme called lipoxygenase to form hydroperoxy acids or peroxides. This process is similar to the oxidation that takes place to such acids left unprotected by antioxidants in the air outside the body. Hydroperoxy acids are highly undesirable since they are toxic to membranes and cells in a manner akin to rancidity in exposed fats. Hence any nutrient that prevents overproduction of hydroperoxy acids, either directly or through the enzyme that produces them, would be expected to be beneficial to health.

In two important papers from Ohio State University, D. Cornwell (1979) and E. T. Gwebu (1980) have reported that vitamin E inhibits the platelet enzyme lipoxygenase in rabbits. Platelets from rabbits supplemented with vitamin E had much less lipoxygenase activity than platelets from vitamin E-deficient or normal rabbits. Extension of the studies to human platelets indicated that preincubation with the vitamin reduced the enzyme activity significantly. The importance of this finding was emphasized in Cornwell's paper; his studies suggest that the proliferation of smooth muscle cells of the aorta is controlled in part by the oxidant stress supplied by the hydroperoxy fatty acids produced by the enzyme lipoxygenase. Rapidly proliferating cells are resistant to peroxidation and hence desirable, and vitamin E stimulates cell proliferation by inhibiting the enzyme. This in turn prevents the formation of a fatty streak in the aorta which is a prerequisite of atherogenic plaque formation.

Hydroperoxy fatty acids are undesirable in other ways, according to publications by W. Forster (1980). These compounds actually inhibit the action of prostacyclin, the "good" hormone that prevents platelet aggregation. Hence any factor that reduces the level of hydroperoxy fatty acids will enable prostacyclin to function effectively. Forster was unable to show a direct effect of vitamin E upon prostacyclin synthesis, but what he did demonstrate in his experimental rabbits was that pretreatment with vitamin E 1) inhibited the enzyme lipoxygenase and hence the formation of hydroperoxy acids and 2) inhibited the formation of the "bad" hormone thromboxane. Beneficial effects of vitamin E on inhibition of thrombus formation must therefore lie with its ability to prevent excessive production of the "bad" prostaglandin and its removal of the substances that inhibit the "good" prostaglandin.

Other reports have studied the effect of intravenous arachidonic acid on the blood of rabbits. This acid is a potent platelet aggregating agent and when injected into the bloodstream of the rabbit it causes vasoconstriction and massive thrombus formations in the blood vessels and organs, killing the animal. Presumably the effect is due to a combination of overproduction of hydroperoxy acids which inhibit prostacyclin, and excessive synthesis of thromboxane. We thus have a useful test system to study the effect of antithrombotic drugs.

M. Barrett and S. O'Regan (1980) used this test system to study the effect of vitamin E. When the vitamin, at an intravenous dose of 150 mg/kg body weight, was given five minutes before the lethal dose of arachidonic acid, it prevented death of the rabbits. There was no deposition of thrombi or blood clots in the organs where they would be expected from injection of arachidonic acid alone. They suggest that "vitamin E succeeds in arresting and inhibiting completely the pathological cascade initiated by arachidonic acid infusion."

Much effort is at present being put into ways of stabilizing prostacyclin so that it can be used as a drug to prevent and treat thrombosis and related diseases. There are already some clinical reports indicating that prostacyclin is beneficial in the successful therapy of advanced arteriosclerosis. However, because of its instability the prostaglandin had to be infused into the bloodstream continuously for three days. Nevertheless the patients involved continued to derive clinical benefit for a further six weeks (A. Szczeklik et al., 1979). All of the studies on vitamin E suggest that it is a natural substance that can exert the same beneficial effects as prostacyclin. How much simpler it is to ensure an adequate daily intake of the vitamin throughout life.

Atherosclerosis. Atherosclerosis is a complex and multifactorial disorder which implies the presence of multiple risk factors. No matter what the cause, however, the end result is an invasion of the inner blood vessel wall by fats and cholesterol resulting in the deposition of atheromatous plaques. These plaques decrease the elasticity of the blood vessel wall and also thicken, reducing the width of the blood vessel and restricting blood flow. Not all atheromatous plaques contain cholesterol but it is generally believed that a high blood cholesterol is more conducive to their development.

Before we look at the therapeutic role of vitamin E in preventing and treating atherosclerosis it is necessary to review what we know about blood cholesterol. At a Washington symposium on March 24, 1981, Dr. Bryan Brewer of the National Heart, Lung and Blood Institute reported on the role of dietary cholesterol and fat in the development of heart disease. In the United States heart attacks occur every twenty seconds and are a major cause of death. Factors in premature heart attack (before age sixty-five) include high blood pressure, high blood cholesterol levels and smoking. Risk increases from low to high levels of these factors in a smooth progression.

Cholesterol is a fatty substance with distinct biochemical functions that are essential to the working of the body. Triglycerides are fats and oils containing three fatty acids, each of which may be saturated or unsaturated, combined with glycerol. Cholesterol and triglycerides cannot be dissolved or transported as such in plasma. They are carried by proteins and the protein-fat complex is called a lipoprotein. It is the way in which cholesterol and fats are carried in the plasma that determines to a large extent whether they are likely to be deposited on the blood vessel walls or not.

The four major groups of lipoproteins are characterized by density and size. They may be thought of as globules ranging from big light globules down to small heavy ones. The largest are called chylomicrons and this is the form in which fat is absorbed from the diet. The next two smaller globules are known as Very Low Density Lipoproteins (VLDL) and Low Density Lipoproteins (LDL). The smallest and most dense globules are called High Density Lipoproteins (HDL). Each lipoprotein has a particular function but the important feature is the proportion of each that is present in plasma.

When cholesterol and triglycerides are eaten, they are reduced to small globule size (chylomicrons) and transported from the intestine to the liver. In the liver they are transferred to VLDL, then transported from that organ to other parts of the body. However, those destined for muscle cells are transported there by LDL. The reverse process from body cells back to the liver involves carriage by HDL. The only way excess cholesterol in the body can be disposed of is by the liver. This organ converts it to bile salts, which are eventually excreted via the bile and feces.

High plasma cholesterol is a risk factor for coronary heart disease but the risk is primarily associated with LDL. In contrast, HDL has a protective effect against heart disease. Hence HDL is the "good" form of cholesterol, probably because high levels of it result in a more efficient removal of excess body cholesterol from body cells.

Vitamin E can influence cholesterol metabolism in two ways. First, it appears to actually decrease blood cholesterol levels. Second, it can alter the proportion of the various density lipoproteins to favor an increase in the good HDL. The animal model for studying cholesterol metabolism is usually the rabbit and many studies have indicated a beneficial effect of vitamin E.

Typical is the report by R. B. Wilson et al. (1978), who compared vitamin E with synthetic antioxidants. Rabbits were fed an atherosclerosis-producing diet consisting of high butter intakes. There were three groups of animals on the diet: one group received supplementary vitamin E (equivalent to 400 IU per day in humans); a second group was given BHA (butylated hydroxyanisole), a synthetic antioxidant much used in foods and drugs; and the third group were fed the basal diet. After three years on the diets it was found that aortic and coronary atherosclerosis were less frequent and extensive in rabbits supplemented with vitamin E than in those fed the basal diet or the one supplemented with BHA. Measurement of blood levels of cholesterol over the three years indicated that these were lower in the vitamin E-treated animals. Prevention of hypercholesterolemia was regarded as the main factor in inhibiting atherosclerosis.

Human studies confirming the effect of vitamin E in reducing blood cholesterol levels were reported by M. Passeri and U. Butturini, of the University of Parma, Italy, in a 1981 international symposium in Madrid. They point out, however, that although vitamin E alone has this beneficial effect at the 300–400 IU per day intake, a synergistic action with adequate intakes of vitamin A and C is probably more efficient.

A personal report by Dr. W. J. Hermann (1980) claims that when he took 600 IU of d-alpha tocopherol acetate (natural vitamin E) daily for thirty days, the proportion of HDL cholesterol in his blood plasma increased dramatically from 9 percent to 40 percent. He then repeated this dosage regime on ten volunteers, five of whom had normal blood plasma lipoprotein profiles and five who had low HDL cholesterol levels. After one month's supplementation with daily 600 IU of vitamin E there was a change in the proportion of HDL cholesterol present. The normal group showed a 50 percent increase in HDL cholesterol, but most significant was the 200 percent increase in the proportion of HDL cholesterol in the other group. In no case was there a significant change in total plasma cholesterol.

These findings were not confirmed in another study, reported by L. Hatam and H. Kayden (1981). These researchers found no effect of vitamin E on the distribution of cholesterol in various lipoproteins but they were using different analytical techniques. The main objection to this study was in the choice of subjects, over half of whom had higher than normal HDL cholesterol levels anyway, so that any increase in them would be minimal. Differences in subject age and the prevalence of obesity may also account for the variations in response in both studies.

Further studies from other groups that were reported in 1982 also give variable results, indicating that there is no clearcut conclusion to be drawn about the beneficial effect of vitamin E on HDL cholesterol levels. Joseph J. Barboriak (1982), from the Medical College of Wisconsin, gave forty-three subjects a total of 800 IU of alpha tocopherol daily for four weeks. Male patients with spinal cord injuries were included, since as a group such patients have low HDL cholesterol levels. Some of the men who were joggers or long-distance runners had unusually high initial levels of HDL cholesterol, while others had low levels. Administration of vitamin E for four weeks "resulted in a statistically significant increase of plasma HDL cholesterol levels" in men who had low initial levels and in women. The levels decreased after vitamin E was discontinued. The results were claimed to have "confirmed the initial report by Hermann (1980) that the effect of alpha tocopherol is primarily seen in subjects with low initial HDL cholesterol levels."

Donald R. Howard (1982) from the Maine Medical Center claimed he was unable to repeat the beneficial effects of vitamin E reported by Hermann. A total of thirty-nine normal volunteers were given 600 IU of dl-alpha tocopherol daily for thirty days. There was no significant change in HDL cholesterol. As in previous studies, it looks as if differences in response to vitamin E may be explained by variation in the choice of subjects for study. Normal, healthy subjects are likely to have the right proportion of HDL cholesterol in their plasma; therefore vitamin E is unlikely to change this significantly. It is only where there is a prevalence of the LDL cholesterol that the vitamin is likely to redress the balance in favor of HDL cholesterol.

It is highly probable that vitamin E is not the only factor that determines the proportion of the "good" HDL cholesterol in the blood. Other experiments (F. Yokata, 1981) indicate that in vitamin C deficiency, the level of HDL cholesterol is low. Once vitamin C is given there is a dramatic increase in HDL cholesterol. Hence any trial where only one factor is studied in isolation may give variable results. The moral of this work seems to ensure an adequate intake of vitamin E to keep HDL cholesterol levels up but at the same time make certain that vitamin C and vitamin A intakes are sufficient for complete inhibition of atherosclerosis.

Although we should therefore aim at increasing the proportion of HDL cholesterol in the blood, it must be remembered that low density lipoproteins have other functions and that they are essential, albeit in lower concentration. When low density lipoproteins are absent the result is a rare hereditary disease called abetalipoproteinemia or acanthocytosis. This is related to very low levels of vitamin E in the blood, due mainly to malabsorption. Growth failure is prominent in childhood. In adolescence neurological abnormality results in progressive disability. Death may occur in early adult life, usually from cardiac involvement. There is no medical treatment available.

However, a report by E. Azizi et al. (1978) offers some hope to those suffering from the disease. An eleven-year-old girl with the disease was treated with vitamins A and E via the intramuscular route, once a week for two and a half years. This was essential because of the inability of the child to absorb the vitamins from the intestinal system.

Some improvements in the neurological and visual deficiencies were noted. In the words of the authors, "On changing to oral vitamin E and later with addition of medium chain triglycerides (simple fats) to the diet, a considerable improvement in general wellbeing, neuromuscular lesions and ophthalmological symptoms was noted." At the time of the report this regime had lasted for sixty-seven months and the condition of the girl was regarded as stable.

Thrombophlebitis. Thrombophlebitis is most simply defined as a thrombus in a vein surrounded by an area of inflammation. Although usually occurring in the legs, it is possible for bits of the thrombus to break off and lodge in the arteries of the lung. The resulting pulmonary embolism then becomes a life threatening situation. Surgery is one of the main stimulants of thrombi; therefore their prevention during any operative procedure becomes of prime importance. Vitamin E has long been advocated as the simplest and most efficient tool in preventing thrombus formation.

One of the main proponents for the prevention of thromboembolic disease by vitamin E is Dr. Alton Ochsner (1968) who stated: "For 15 years I have used alpha tocopherol routinely in the treatment of patients who have been subjected to trauma of any magnitude. None of these patients have had pulmonary embolism." His supplementary regime consisted of giving between 200 and 600 IU of alpha tocopherol daily, either by intramuscular injection or by mouth, beginning no later than the day of surgery (but preferably before) and continuing through the post-operative period. In addition calcium gluconate was given intravenously (10 ml of a 10 percent solution every twenty-four or forty-eight hours). The calcium was an essential part of the treatment.

In a later publication, Drs. J. D. and P. B. Kanofsky (1981) reviewed six clinical trials from American and British literature that compared vitamin E-calcium-treated groups with controls in the prevention of thrombi. None used a double-blind design, which meant that there was the possibility of diagnosis of deep vein thrombosis or pulmonary embolism by clinicians who may have been influenced by bias. Nevertheless, the authors concluded that in the control groups, failure to use the vitamin E-calcium treatment doubled the risk of peripheral venous thrombosis; increased the risk of pulmonary embolism six-fold; and increased the chances of fatal pulmonary embolism ninefold. It is believed that vitamin E has this beneficial effect because, as we have seen previously, it appears to inhibit platelet aggregation—an important factor in the formation of a thrombus. Experimental evidence has come from studies on pigs, where inadequate levels of vitamin E were found to induce the formation of vascular thrombosis.

Dr. H. J. Roberts (1978) has refuted the alleged beneficial action of vitamin E in suppressing thrombosis. He has noted that in ten years of patient observation, forty-six individuals who were taking high doses (i.e., more than 400 IU daily) of alpha tocopherol had suspected or diagnosed thrombophlebitis. The symptoms of this complaint included discomfort of the lower limbs, with or without edema, and tenderness in the calves and thighs. These complaints disappeared when vitamin E supplementation was stopped and reappeared in two cases when vitamin E was resumed. Pulmonary embolism was confirmed as highly suspect in 57 percent of the patients.

He concludes that vitamin E may encourage thrombosis in patients who already have metabolic cardiovascular or hormonal disorders which predispose to small-vessel disease, platelet aggregation and thrombosis, especially if estrogens (as for example in the contraceptive pill) are being taken.

There could be a number of reasons for these opposing claims for the connection between vitamin E and thrombophlebitis. Roberts was merely making observations on patients who claimed to take vitamin E; the trials reported by Kanofsky were controlled studies. The latter trials also used calcium along with the vitamin E, and this mineral could have played an important role.

It may also be expected that in view of the widespread use of high doses of tocopherol in the world, its adverse effects should occur more often than they do.

VITAMIN E AS A THERAPEUTIC AGENT

Anemia. One of the few generally recognized uses for vitamin E is in the treatment of hemolytic anemia in premature babies. Hemolytic anemia is characterized by a shortened life of the red blood cell and an increased tendency for this to burst. Once the contents have been released, the hemoglobin is unable to function as an oxygen carrier and the number of red blood cells available is reduced, resulting in the typical symptoms of anemia. A consequence of the shortened survival time of red blood cells in preterm infants is an increase in the blood level of bilirubin. This is a bile pigment which is an excretion product from the disposal of hemoglobin and in excess it leads to jaundice of the newborn. Bilirubinemia is usually treated in babies by phototherapy, exposing the child to special sources of light until the level of bilirubin is reduced to normal levels. It is not clear how such phototherapy functions. However, S. J. Gross (1979) has studied some forty infants, some of whom were under 1500 grams in weight, and has shown that administering vitamin E during the first three days of life enabled the time of phototherapy to be reduced from an average of 107 hours to only 48.

There is a poor transfer of vitamin E from mother to fetus across the placenta so that both premature and full-term newborn babies may have relatively low levels of vitamin E in both tissues and blood. The blood plasma levels of the vitamin in newborn infants average about 5 mg/liter, which is only half that found in normal adults.

The need for supplemental vitamin E in the newborn has been widely recognized, particularly in the premature infant. Human milk is sufficiently rich in vitamin E to satisfy the baby's needs but cow's milk, frequently used in bottle feeding, contains much smaller amounts. There are numerous studies indicating that vitamin E reduces the hemolysis of the red blood cells of preterm infants (e.g., Graeber, Williams and Oski, 1977). However, recent clinical trials have shown that even in adults certain types of hemolytic anemia respond favorably to vitamin E treatment. This represents a significant step forward in the therapy of an hitherto incurable disease.

Two rare hereditary red blood cell disorders, glutathione synthetase deficiency and chronic hemolytic glucose-6-phosphate dehydrogenase deficiency, are characterized by compromised intracellular reductive capacity and decreased red blood cell survival. The first named condition is thought to result from inadequate glutathione synthesis during oxidative stress leading to denaturation of hemoglobin and premature removal of affected red blood cells. In the second condition there is lowered production of reduced nicotinamide adenine dinucleotide phosphate (NADPH), leading in turn to decreases in glutathione synthesis, so the end result is similar in both hereditary diseases. Vitamin E in high oral doses (800 IU per day) improved red blood cell survival in both of these disorders. Hence a similar trial was performed with twenty-three patients suffering from Mediterranean glucose-6-phosphate dehydrogenase deficiency and reported by L. Corash and colleagues (1980) and F. A. Oski (1980).

Three months of vitamin E administration at the dosage of four 200 mg chewable tablets given at one time resulted in decreased chronic hemolysis as evidenced by improved red-cell life span, increased hemoglobin concentration of the blood and decreased reticulocystosis (a measure of red cell production) as compared to base line values. "Evaluation after one year of vitamin E administration demonstrated sustained improvement in all these indices." Further evidence is required of longer term administration of vitamin E in these disorders, especially the effects at times of hemolytic crises, to determine whether vitamin E has a therapeutic role in this group of blood disorders, but preliminary results are encouraging. Confirmation has now come from European studies.

A related anemia is beta thalassemia or Mediterranean anemia. It is a congenital anemia occurring in populations from countries bordering the Mediterranean and from southeast Asia and it is characterized by defective hemoglobin synthesis and by ineffective red blood cell formation. Heterozygous beta thalassemia is known as thalassemia minor and is usually asymptomatic, but typical symptoms occur in homozygotes (thalassemia major). In thalassemia major low serum alpha tocopherol levels are usually found. Treatment with the vitamin results in increased blood levels, decreased lipid peroxidation and in some cases prolonged red blood cell survival (Rachilewitz, Shifter and Kahane, 1980).

The treatment of thalassemia minor with vitamin E was reported by R. Miniero and associates (1981) from the University of Turin, Italy at a recent international symposium. Ten patients were evaluated to determine if vitamin E could reduce oxidative stress and improve anemia. For three months each patient received between 400 and 600 IU vitamin E daily by mouth. In half of them biochemical parameters showed a reduction of lipid peroxidation and increased red blood cell survival. These encouraging results are being used as a basis for a larger scale study of the benefits of vitamin E in treating beta thalassemia.

There is also preliminary evidence that vitamin E can help in treating sickle-cell anemia. D. Chiv and B. Lubin (1979) found that patients with this disorder have low levels of vitamin E in their blood plasma and red cells. These people appear to have an increased susceptibility of their red blood cells to peroxidation which was corrected in *in vitro* experiments by vitamin E. Confirmation that treating patients with sickle-cell anemia with 450 IU of dl-alpha tocopherol daily reduced the number of irreversibly sickled cells that were circulating comes from studies reported by C. L. Natta (1980). The number of sickle cells in the bloodstream is related to the extent of hemolysis of the blood, so any reduction is beneficial. Prolonged administration of vitamin E is now being investigated to see if it will alleviate other aspects of the clinical condition as a result of a reduction in circulating sickle cells.

The prevention of blindness in babies. Very small premature babies commonly have immature lungs; this leads to respiratory distress, and therefore they have to be nursed in an oxygen rich incubator if they are to survive. Without sufficient oxygen the infant's brain may suffer irreversible damage. With too much oxygen another complication may develop—damage to the blood vessels in the eyes. The condition is called retrolental fibroplasia which, when severe, can lead to permanent blindness. It is the direct result of an oxidative stress.

The connection between excess oxygen and retrolental fibroplasia has been recognized for thirty years but as neonatal medicine has improved, the result has been a higher survival rate among the smallest babies, with a consequent increased risk of developing the condition. Despite a number of research studies it is impossible to recommend a safe level of oxygen for these infants.

Vitamin E, because of its antioxidant properties, would appear to be a natural therapeutic agent for the condition and it has been tried over the last thirty years with variable results. Twenty-five years separate two of the best controlled studies (W. C. and E. V. Owens, 1949, and L. Johnson, D. Schaffer and T. R. Boggs, 1974). Both sets of investigators concluded that there was a relationship between the prevention of retrolental fibroplasia and the administration of vitamin E as a prophylactic agent. Two recent studies appear to confirm the effectiveness of vitamin E in this respect.

P. Gunby (1980) reported in the *Journal of the American Medical Association* that high doses of vitamin E appear to result in a reduction in overall incidence of retrolental fibroplasia and a decrease in both the severity and duration of acute stage disease. Healing appears also to be favorably influenced.

The most comprehensive study was reported in the *New England Journal of Medicine* in December 1981 by Dr. Helen Hittner and her collaborators from Baylor College of Medicine and the College of Optometry, University of Houston. They performed a double-blind study (i.e., neither patient nor doctor knows which individuals are being treated) on 101 preterm infants who weighed less than 1500 grams at birth. These infants had respiratory distress and survived at least four weeks. Two groups were studied. A control group of 51 infants received 5 mg per kilogram body weight of vitamin E per day by mouth. Fifty infants received 100 mg per kilogram body weight of the vitamin also by mouth. The first dose of vitamin E in every case was given within the first twenty-four hours of life and then daily while in the hospital. Synthetic vitamin E (dl-alpha tocopherol) was used throughout. The state of the retina was evaluated in every child during the third week of life and weekly thereafter. Retrolental fibroplasia was scored on a classification from Grade I (neovascularization of the retina) through

Grade IV (retinal detachment), although none were allowed to proceed beyond Grade II without surgical treatment, and none reached Grade IV.

The results of the trial were highly encouraging. There was a significant decrease in the incidence of retrolental fibroplasia in those receiving 100 mg vitamin E per kilogram body weight and none proceeded to Grade III of the disease. When multivariate analysis was applied to both control and treatment groups, the severity of retrolental fibroplasia was found to be significantly reduced in infants given the higher dose of vitamin E.

The researchers conclude that their data indicate that vitamin E does not eliminate the occurrence of mild to moderate grades of retrolental fibroplasia. However, it should be regarded as part of the clinician's armamentarium which can be used to diminish severity of the condition and hence reduce blindness secondary to the disorder. Their advice is not to withhold vitamin E until after oxygen has been given, since early administration of the vitamin allows blood plasma levels to build up and confer protection upon ocular tissue. Sometimes even greater intakes of the vitamin may be justified.

Cystic breast disease. About 20 percent of American women suffer from noncancerous lumps in the breast tissue known popularly as cysts and clinically as fibrocystic breast disease, mammary dysplasia or fibrous mastopathy. Women with at least some types of fibrocystic breast disease are thought to be at a twofold to eightfold greater risk of developing breast cancer. Even those whose lumps remain benign often experience some discomfort.

As long ago as 1965, reports had come from the Boston University School of Medicine (A. A. Abrams) that moderate to complete relief of premenstrual symptoms in sixteen patients with fibrocystic breast disease had been achieved with vitamin E taken orally. Palpable softening of the breasts and a reduction in cyst size were the benefits noted in thirteen other patients when given vitamin E. Later studies carried out at Baltimore's Sinai Hospital confirmed these results, claiming that vitamin E relieved breast tenderness, caused cyst regression and on a biochemical note altered adrenal steroid hormone excretion in twenty women (R. S. London, 1978).

A double-blind clinical trial on the use of vitamin E in relieving cystic breast disease has recently been reported by the same Baltimore group headed by R. S. London (1980). Twenty-six patients and eight control subjects were treated with a placebo for four weeks, followed by 600 IU of vitamin E daily for eight weeks. Various blood hormone levels were measured in an attempt to learn whether the vitamin's action is mediated through hormone synthesis or alteration of lipoproteins. All subjects were between twenty-three and forty years old (average thirty-four years) and all were diagnosed as suffering from middle-stage mammary dysplasia.

At the end of the test period ten patients showed a good response, twelve were regarded as fair responders and four gained no benefit. A good response meant that the disease regressed. The lumps went away and the individuals noticed tremendous clinical improvements. Significant relief in 85 percent of the patients studied is an encouraging clinical response but hormone changes were also noted.

The vitamin had profound effects in reducing to normal the elevated hormone levels found in most women who have cysts. Since increased amounts of certain hormones have been linked to breast cancer in older women, reducing those levels with vitamin E may possibly prevent cancer from developing. In the women who responded there were other beneficial biochemical changes. Cholesterol carried as High Density Lipoprotein increased and, as we have already seen, this response is thought to give protection from cardiovascular disease.

On the basis of his findings Dr. London recommends that clinicians should try vitamin E as a first-line treatment for benign cystic breast disease. "I think our work highly suggests that vitamin E is effective in these patients," he says. "We found absolutely no side effects in terms of clinical derangements, and it worked in a high percentage of patients. If the clinicians can get symptomatic relief in patients with something as benign as vitamin E, I think it's a reasonable therapy."

Vitamin E may also help as a therapy for breast cancer. Dr. London (1981) has extended his studies on cystic breast disease treatment with vitamin E to postulate that the vitamin's effect on blood steroid hormones may reduce the future risk of breast cancer in the individual. Patients who develop breast cancer have an abnormal pattern of the steroid hormones estradiol, estriol and progesterone in the blood plasma long before the clinical disease manifests itself. In a double-blind study, 88 percent of the seventeen patients treated with 600 IU per day of alpha tocopherol showed clinical response to the therapy. There was also a statistically significant rise in the ratio of progesterone to estradiol in those patients with cancer. This ratio is usually abnormally low in this disease. Redressing the balance of hormones with vitamin E could therefore represent a significant step in the prevention and treatment of breast cancer.

Resistance to disease. It has been reported by Tanaka, Fujiwara and Torisu (1979) that vitamin E enhances resistance to bacterial infection. The evidence by these authors came from studies on mice where the effects of the vitamin on the humoral immune response were studied. Mice were fed a diet supplemented with 0, 20 and 200 mg of vitamin E as alpha tocopheryl acetate per kilogram of food. Using standard immunological tests, it was shown that the antibody response is augmented by dietary supplementation with vitamin E. The study confirmed previous investigations from other research groups in which chickens were given increased protection against E. coli by vitamin E supplementation.

Similar studies on human beings point to an important role for vitamin E in the defense against bacterial infection. The main line of this defense resides in the white blood cells, which have the ability to move toward and engulf microorganisms or foreign bodies that appear in the blood. This process is known as phagocytosis. An important pointer to the role of vitamin E in white blood cells was provided by L. Hatam and H. Kayden (1979), who have reported that normal white blood cells have about thirty times as much vitamin E as red blood cells.

An important collaborative study from several prestigious institutes has shown for the first time that the white blood cells of human beings may be involved in vitamin E physiology (L.A. Boxer and Associates, 1979). In glutathione synthetase deficiency some of the white blood cells become deficient in glutathione, which in one form is needed to dispose of the toxic hydrogen peroxide. A patient with an impaired ability to synthesize glutathione had suffered frequent bouts of ear infection during the first two years of his life. He was treated with

400 IU of vitamin E daily for three months, after which he had no further episodes of bacterial infection for the next eighteen months. His brother, who had also inherited glutathione synthetase deficiency, was treated with vitamin E from the fourth day of his life and he has remained free of infection while on this therapy.

These are preliminary studies and the relationship of vitamin E to other factors that influence the immune response, for example vitamin C, has to be worked out, but they do appear to represent yet another function of this versatile vitamin in maintaining good health.

NEW INSIGHT INTO VITAMIN E POTENCY

Vitamin E occurs naturally and when it does, it is referred to as d-alpha tocopherol. However, d-alpha tocopherol rarely occurs alone and it is usually accompanied by d-beta tocopherol, d-gamma tocopherol and d-delta tocopherol. All of these differ slightly in chemical structure but there are gross differences in their biological activity. If d-alpha tocopherol is regarded as 100 percent, the d-beta, d-gamma and d-delta forms are 40 percent, 8 percent and 1 percent respectively when measured in the female rat resorption test. Nature is therefore very selective in her production of the E vitamins but the synthetic chemist is not so fortunate. He is unable to make the d-form exclusively when synthesizing the vitamin in the laboratory; thus the end result is a mixture of the biologically active d-forms and the biologically useless l-forms. Not surprisingly, on a milligram for milligram basis, natural vitamin E as d-alpha tocopherol is more active biologically than the synthesized dl-alpha tocopherol. Hence for many years, based on animal testing, 1 milligram of synthetic dl-alpha tocopheryl acetate was assigned a biological potency of 1 IU and a milligram of the more active d-alpha tocopheryl acetate was regarded as equivalent to 1.36 IU, that is, some 36 percent more potent. The free form d-alpha tocopherol, which is rarely used as a supplement because it is less stable than the acetate, was found to be 49 percent more active than synthetic dl-alpha tocopheryl acetate. The difference in spelling—tocopherol or tocopheryl—depends on whether the word is followed by the ester—acetate or succinate—in which case the "yl" form is used.

In recent years the potency of the commercially available dl-alpha tocopheryl acetate has been questioned. When the original international unit standard was established the tocopheryl acetate was prepared from an entirely synthetic ring (chroman) and a natural (isoprenoid) side chain. One milligram of the acetate of this partially synthetic tocopherol (known as 2-ambo-alpha tocopheryl acetate) was ascribed the biological potency of 1 IU. It was at the time generally called dl-alpha tocopheryl acetate although this name should really be properly given to the present-day commercially available compound (known as all-rac alpha tocopheryl acetate) which is entirely synthetic both in the side chain and in the chroman ring. Until recently challenged, this latter form has automatically been considered to have the same biological potency as the "2-ambo" semisynthetic form, i.e., 1 mg to 1 IU.

S. A. Ames (1979) has looked at the problem and compared the biological potencies of the two forms of dl-tocopheryl acetates in the rat test. His results show considerable differences between them. If the original standard 2-ambo-alpha tocopheryl acetate is given a value of 1.00, then the natural d-alpha tocopheryl acetate has a relative potency in the long-accepted rat fetal resorption assay of 1.66. This is considerably higher than the currently accepted value of 1.36. Preparations of the modern material all-rac alpha tocopheryl acetate similarly compared had a relative potency of 0.81. When this was standardized against the natural d-alpha tocopheryl acetate, it had a relative potency of only 0.52. What it all means is that in this test at least, all synthetic vitamin E acetate is only half as active as the natural material.

These results led M. K. Horwitt (1980) to study how active the various preparations of vitamin E were in human beings. Vitamin E-depleted subjects (all males) were given supplements of the various tocopheryl acetates for 138 days and the blood levels were measured. Daily doses of 7.5 mg, 15 mg, 60 mg and 240 mg of natural d-alpha tocopheryl acetate were compared with 10 mg, 20 mg, 80 mg and 320 mg of the synthetic variety of the vitamins. When evaluated he found that all-rac alpha tocopheryl acetate (modern synthetic material) may have no more than half the biological potency of the natural d-alpha tocopheryl acetate when used as a supplement in E-depleted subjects. On the basis of these studies, which confirm those of Ames, Horwitt suggests that present-day synthetic vitamin E should be allotted only half the biological potency of the natural form of the vitamin (d-alpha tocopheryl acetate) when calculating human requirements. The previously accepted figure was 74 percent.

These conclusions by Horwitt stimulated other studies on the relative potencies of semisynthetic vitamin E acetate and all-synthetic vitamin E acetate and two papers provide contrary evidence. The first was from L. Machlin and M. Brin (1981) of Hoffman-la Roche, New Jersey, and their results were based on the curative effects of vitamin E on muscle dystrophy in E-deprived rats. They found that the 2-ambo-alpha tocopheryl acetate partially synthetic form displays only 92 percent of the activity of the all-rac alpha tocopheryl acetate completely synthetic form. They concluded that both were substantially the same, so that modern synthetic vitamin E acetate may be regarded as having 74 percent of the potency of the natural material.

H. Weiser and M. Vecchi (1981) report somewhat different results from Hoffman-la Roche in Basel, Switzerland. They used the rat resorption test and found that the all-rac alpha tocopheryl acetate (all-synthetic) was 9 percent less active than the 2-ambo-alpha tocopheryl Jersey group. They also concluded that there was no statistically significant difference in the two synthetic forms.

These groups differ from Horwitt's conclusions in another way. Horwitt claimed that natural vitamin E is lost from the blood at a slower rate than the synthetic vitamin is. The Hoffman-la Roche teams claimed to demonstrate an equivalent loss of both forms, using the same data. There is of course no guarantee that the relative activities of various tocopherols established by animal experiments are the same as those in man. Additional evaluation in man is therefore considered desirable.

In view of this conflicting evidence, there is little doubt that the safest course in supplementation is to use natural vitamin

E, i.e., d-alpha tocopheryl acetate, whenever possible. On a well-established and generally agreed basis of one milligram of the natural acetate being equivalent to 1.36 IU, a daily dose measured either by weight or by biological potency is simple to calculate.

REFERENCES

Abrams, A. A. 1965. *New Engl. J. Med.* 272:1080.
Ames, S. A. 1979. *J. Nutr.* 109:2198.
Azizi, E., Zaidman, J. L., Eshchar, J. and Szeinberg, A. 1978. *Acton Paediat. Scand.* 67:797.
Barboriak, J. J. 1982. *Amer. J. Clin. Path.* 77:371.
Barrett, M. and O'Regan, S. 1980. *Prostaglandins and Medicine* 5:337.
Binder, H. J. and Shapiro, H. M. 1967. *Amer. J. Clin. Nutr.* 20:594.
Boxer, L. A., Oliver, J. M., Spielberg, S. P., Allen, J. M. and Schulman, H. D. 1979. *New Engl. J. Med.* 301:901.
Chiv, D. and Lubin, B. 1979. *J. Lab. Clin. Med.* 94:542.
Corash, L., Spielberg, S. P., Bartsocas, C., Boxer, L. A., Steinherz, R., Sheetz, M., Egan, M., Schlessleman, J. and Schulman, J. D. 1980. *New Engl. J. Med.* 303:416.
Cornwell, D. 1979. *Lipids* 14:194.
Farrell, P. M., Bieri, J. G., Fratantoni, J. F., Wood, R. E. and Di Sant'Agnese, P. A. 1977. *J. Clin. Invest.* 60:233.
Forster, W. 1980. *Acta Med. Scand.* (Suppl.) 642:47, 35.
Graeber, J. E., Williams, M. L. and Oski, F. A. 1977. *J. Pediat.* 90:282.
Gross, S. J. 1979. *Pediatrics* 64:321.
Gunby, P. 1980. *J. Amer. Med. Assoc.* 243:1021, 1025.
Gwebu, E. T. 1980. *Res. Comm. in Chemical Pathology and Pharmacology* 28:361.
Haeger, K. 1974. *Amer. J. Clin. Nutr.* 27:1179.
Hatam, L. and Kayden, H. 1979. *J. Lipid Res.* 20:639.
Hatam, L. and Kayden, H. 1981. *Amer. J. Clin. Path.* 76:122.

Hermann, W. J., Ward, K. and Faucett, J. 1979. *Amer. J. Clin. Path.* 72:848.

Hittner, H. M., Godio, L. B., Rudolph, A. J., Adams, J. M., Garcia-Prats, J. A., Friedman, Z., Kautz, J. A. and Monaco, W. A. 1981. *New Engl. J. Med.* 305:1365.

Horwitt, M. K. 1980. *Amer. J. Clin. Nutr.* 33:1856.

Howard, D. R. 1982. *Amer. J. Clin. Path.* 77:86.

Johnson, L., Schaffer, D. and Boggs, T. R. 1974. *Amer. J. Clin. Nutr.* 27:1158.

Kanofsky, J. D. and Kanofsky, P. B. 1981. *New Engl. J. Med.* July 16, 1973.

London, R. S. 1978. *Breast* 4:19.

London, R. S., Sundaram, G. S., Schultz, M., Naier, P. P. and Goldstein, P. 1980. *J. Amer. Med. Assoc.* 244:1077.

London, R. S. 1981. *Cancer Research* 41:3811.

Machlin, L. and Brin, M. 1981. *Amer. J. Clin. Nutr.* 34:1633.

Miniero, R., Canducci, E., Ghigo, D., Saracco, P. and Vullo, C. 1981. 1st Europ. Symp. on Vitamins. New Aspects in Prevention and Therapy.

Natta, C. L. 1980. *Amer. J. Clin. Nutr.* 33:968.

Ochsner, A. 1968. *Postgrad. Med.* 44:91.

Oski, F. A. 1980. *New Engl. J. Med.* 303:454.

Owens, W. C. and Owens, E. V. 1949. *Amer. J. Ophthalmol.* 32:1631.

Passeri, M. and Butturini, U. 1981. 1st Europ. Symp. on Vitamins. New Aspects in Prevention and Therapy.

Rachilewitz, E. A., Shifter, A. and Kahane, I. 1980. Haematology Service, Hadassah Univ. Hosp. and Biomembrane Res. Lab. Hebrew Univ., Hadassah Med. School, Jerusalem.

Roberts, H. J. 1978. *Lancet*, January 7, 49.

Roberts, H. J. 1981. *J. Amer. Med. Assoc.* 246:129.

Szczeklik, A., Skawinski, S., Gluszko, P., Nizankowski, R., Szczeklik, J. and Gryglewski, R. J. 1979. *Lancet*, May 26.

Tanaka, J., Fujiwara, H. and Torisu, M. 1979. *Immunology* 38:727.

Weiser, H. and Vecchi, M. 1981. *Int. J. Vit. and Nutr. Res.* 51:100.

Wilson, R. B., Middleton, C. C. and Sun, G. Y. 1978. *J. Nutr.* 108:67.

Yokata, F. 1981. *Atherosclerosis* 38:249.